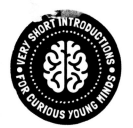

VERY SHORT INTRODUCTIONS • FOR CURIOUS YOUNG MINDS •

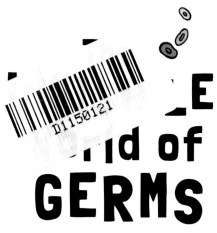

...E
rid of
GERMS

Isabel Thomas

RD
PRESS

Acknowledgements

The publisher and authors would like to
thank the following for permission to use
photographs and other copyright material:

Cover artwork: Geraldine Sy and
Ana Seixas; photos: Shutterstock
and author. **Inside artwork:** Photos:
1(tl): Pavlo S/Shutterstock; p6: Ljupco
Smokovski/Shutterstock; p11: Prachaya
Roekdeethaweesab/Shutterstock;
p16: Wellcome Collection; p18: Oleg
Golovnev/Shutterstock; p19: Prachaya
Roekdeethaweesab/Shutterstock; p21:
Wellcome Collection (CC BY 4.0); p22:
Kateryna Kon/Shutterstock; p24(l): Cosmin
Manci/Shutterstock; p24(r): Lebendkulturen.
de/Shutterstock; p32: Henri Koskinen/
Shutterstock; p33(tl): sciencepics/
Shutterstock; p33(tr): Kateryna Kon/
Shutterstock; p33(bl): Science Photo Library/
Alamy Stock Photo; p33(br): Kateryna Kon/
Shutterstock; p34: David Gregory & Debbie
Marshall (CC BY 4.0); p36–37: abu_zeina/

Shutterstock; p39, p79: SCIEPRO/Getty
Images; p44: Somogyi Laszlo/Shutterstock;
p45: MestoSveta/Shutterstock; p46: F8
studio/Shutterstock; p51: Public Domain;
p55: Kateryna Kon/Shutterstock; p56:
Ekaterina Kolomeets/Shutterstock; p60,
p83: HomeArt/Shutterstock; p63: wasanajai/
Shutterstock; p67: Wellcome Collection
(CC BY 4.0); p71: Sebastian Kaulitzki/
Shutterstock; p80: rvlsoft/Shutterstock;
p81(l): windu/Shutterstock; p81(r): gresei/
Shutterstock; p85: K.K.T Madhusanka/
Shutterstock.

Artwork by Aaron Cushley, Ekaterina
Gorelova, Adam Quest, Ana Seixas,
Geraldine Sy, and Raspberry Books.

Every effort has been made to contact
copyright holders of material reproduced
in this book. Any omissions will be rectified
in subsequent printings if notice is given to
the publisher.

Contents

Chapter 1

What Are Germs?

Wherever you go on Earth—from the highest mountain to the driest desert to the deepest, darkest ocean trenches—you will always be surrounded by living things too tiny to see. They are known as **microbes**. Like all living things, microbes spend their time feeding, getting rid of waste, and reproducing.

Some **microbes** can cause harm when they go about their lives on or inside our bodies. We call these harmful microbes 'germs', and describe them as '**pathogenic**'.

People also use the word 'germs' to describe viruses, which are even smaller than microbes. Viruses don't have all the features of living things, but some of them can cause harm when they get inside our bodies.

Main types of germ

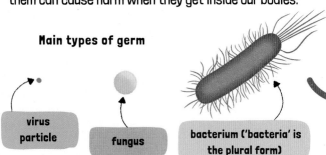

virus particle

fungus

bacterium ('bacteria' is the plural form)

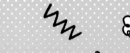

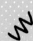

✳ Speak like a scientist ✳

MICROBE

'Micro' means very small, and microbes are the smallest living things. They are so tiny that a single square centimetre of your skin—your fingertip, say—can be home to millions of microbes, but you'll never see them! Most microbes can only be seen with the help of a microscope that can magnify them tens, hundreds, thousands, or even millions of times.

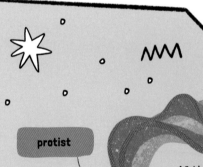

protist

If these germs really were the size they are shown here, you would be **almost six kilometres tall** in comparison!

5

A person with an illness caused by germs is said to have an **infection**. There are germs that infect plants and animals too, and even germs that infect microbes!

The infections caused by pathogenic (meaning disease-causing) microbes and viruses harm millions of people, plants, and animals every year. They include some of the world's most dreaded diseases, from malaria to the coronavirus disease Covid-19. This means that germs have a very bad reputation.

Pesky germs!

But not all microbes and viruses are germs that cause disease. Most are completely harmless—or even help to keep us healthy. As doctors and scientists get to know microbes better, we're discovering that they are just as varied, remarkable, and important as plants and animals.

We'll never be able to rid the world of microbes and viruses, but we wouldn't want to. They shape our world and everything in it—including **YOU**!

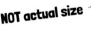

NOT actual size

In this very short introduction to the invisible world of germs, you'll discover that . . .

Scientists figured out that we are walking, talking habitats for tiny living things.

Microbes and viruses like to jump from one living thing to another.

There's a link between gravity and toad vomit.

Viruses get you to do all their work for them.

Doctors use germs to fight germs.

You owe your life to snot, sweat, tears, and earwax!

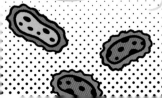

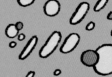

Chapter 2

A Very Short History of Germs

Microbes lived on Earth long before humans. The oldest fossils are found in stromatolites that are around 3.5 billion years old. These rock patterns are only formed when thin layers of microbes get sandwiched by thin layers of sand and silt. This tells us that microbes were the very first living things on the planet.

When a single year between birthdays seems to stretch on forever, it's hard to imagine billions of years. To make it easier, imagine the entire 4.5-billion-year history of planet Earth squashed into the twelve months of a calendar year:

- The first **microbes** appeared in **February**.

- The first plants and animals popped up in **August**.

- The **dinosaurs** died out on **25 December**.

- **Humans** appeared in the last **thirty minutes**.

On this timescale, we only became aware of our tiniest neighbours one second ago! But the clues that we were sharing a planet with microbes were there all along. **Infections** and **infectious diseases** have always been a part of human lives, but it was a long time before anyone worked out that germs were the cause.

When today's doctors examine ancient Egyptian mummies, they can tell that people living 5,000 years ago suffered from tooth decay, colds, malaria, and many other infections that are still common today.

Old ideas

Ancient doctors were brilliant at identifying different diseases, but they had no idea what caused them. Their guesses often involved angry ghosts or ancient gods. An ancient Egyptian, Greek, or Roman doctor was just as likely to prescribe spells as medicines.

real ancient Egyptian remedy

Write the word Abracadabra eleven times, dropping one letter each time. When only the 'A' is left, your illness will have vanished!

The ancient Greeks and Romans worried about plant diseases that destroyed their crops. But they didn't know anything about germs, so they made up stories about angry gods such as Robigus, god of corn. By organizing festivals and offering Robigus gifts, they hoped they could stop the diseases from happening.

Some ancient Greek thinkers came up with different theories. For example, Hippocrates linked diseases to different **fluids** in the body—bile, blood, and snot. He thought diseases happened when these 'humours' got out of balance. This sort of makes sense when you have an uncontrollably runny nose, but his **theory** was wrong. However, people were so desperate to explain and control diseases, even wrong ideas remained popular for hundreds of years.

In the 9th, 10th, and 11th centuries, Islamic doctors such as al-Razi and Ibn Sina studied these ancient ideas. Rather than just accepting what they read, they began carrying out careful observations and experiments of their own. This was the beginning of medicine as a science.

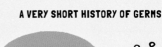

No more spells. I'm going to watch carefully and find out what's really going on!

New ideas

In 1025, Ibn Sina was one of the first people to write about **hygiene** (taking steps to stay clean) and **quarantine** as a way to prevent certain diseases from spreading. But still no one understood why these steps worked so well. So, for hundreds of years, most people believed a mixture of older and newer ideas.

GERM HERO

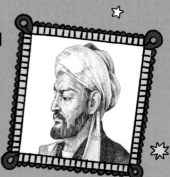

ABU ALI AL-HUSAYN IBN ABD ALLAH IBN SINA

One of the first people to suggest that disease could be caused by living organisms.

For example, in Europe in the Middle Ages, it was common to believe that disease was caused by demons or bad smells. However, during outbreaks of **bubonic plague**, practical steps such as keeping a distance from ill people were used to stop the disease spreading. People understood that they could catch diseases from each other.

Knowing what worked didn't stop people inventing their own 'cures' for bubonic plague. One of the weirdest was invented by Isaac Newton in the 1600s.

He suggested making **lozenges** from a mixture of **dried, powdered toad** and **toad vomit**.

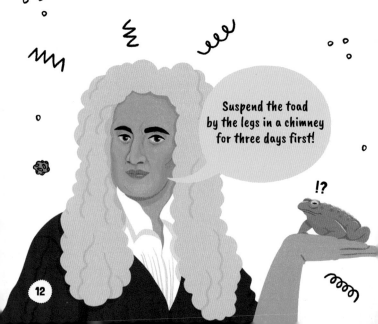

Suspend the toad by the legs in a chimney for three days first!

!?

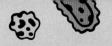

Speak like a scientist

BUBONIC PLAGUE

Bubonic plague is a disease named after one of its symptoms—painful, swollen lymph nodes, or 'buboes'. The disease can kill within days or hours. In the 1300s, there were no treatments and the disease spread quickly as people moved about due to war and trade. Over four years, a pandemic swept through Europe, Asia, and North Africa, killing around one in every three people (at least 25 million people in Europe alone). This terrible pandemic became known as the 'Black Death'.

QUARANTINE

The word quarantine was invented during the Black Death when visitors to the city of Ragusa (now Dubrovnik) were told they had to spend up to forty days on an island before coming into town. 'Quaranta' is Italian for forty. This stopped people spreading the disease before they knew they were ill.

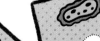

Deadly travellers

War and **trade** spread many more diseases besides bubonic plague (and still do). Some of the most terrible **epidemics** (widespread outbreaks of disease) in history were caused by European explorers travelling to the Americas in the 15th and 16th centuries. They brought smallpox, a horrible infectious disease that spread quickly among Native Americans, including the people of the Aztec and Incan Empires.

The Native Americans had never been exposed to smallpox before—or other nasty European diseases such as measles and mumps. They had no natural immunity (see page 55). After just fifty years, more than 25 million Native Americans had died.

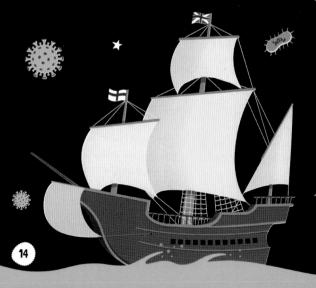

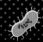

Seeds of disease

At the time, only one person suspected the true cause of these devastating epidemics: an Italian doctor and poet called Girolamo Fracastoro. He came up with the idea that **contagious** diseases were caused by tiny 'seeds' that could multiply quickly. He said they could be transferred from an infected person to other people in three ways—direct contact, on objects such as dirty clothes, or through the air.

This was a **really good** description of germs! But Fracastoro's theory of 1564 didn't catch on, until someone actually saw one of these 'seeds' for the first time.

Following the Middle Ages, Europe exploded with new ideas and inventions, including discoveries about the human body. But it was the invention of the microscope that led to a breakthrough in understanding the cause of infections and infectious diseases.

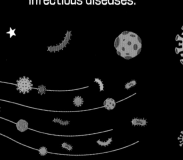

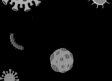

The first microscopes made objects look around ten times bigger, but by the late 1600s, Antonie van Leeuwenhoek was handmaking microscopes that could magnify objects 200 times.

GERM HERO

ANTONIE VAN LEEUWENHOEK

The first person to see microbes and suggest they could be the cause of infectious diseases.

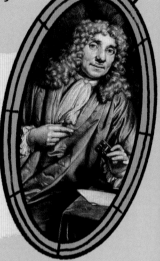

Now he could explore a hidden world beyond his natural senses—and **he was hooked!** Van Leeuwenhoek looked at everything from a **spider's bottom** to a **gnat's eye**.

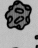

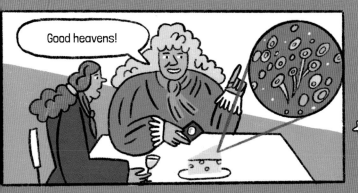

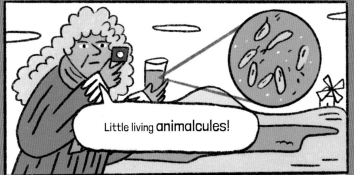

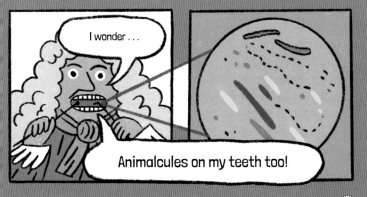

The 'germ' theory of disease

It was another 200 years before Antonie van Leeuwenhoek **was proved right!** Throughout the 1700s and early 1800s, people continued to act on wrong ideas about the causes of disease.

For example, doctors believed that people got fevers because there was too much blood in their body. The 'cure' was to make cuts to let blood out, or even attach leeches to suck blood out!

Things began to change with the work of Louis Pasteur, a French chemist who demonstrated that bacteria were to blame for wine going sour and meat rotting. In 1850, Pasteur carried out experiments that showed microbes did cause disease, at least in caterpillars of silk moths.

GERM HERO

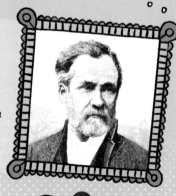

LOUIS PASTEUR

Championed the germ theory of disease and made many other breakthroughs involving microbes.

Evidence came from the world of medicine too. Medics such as Florence Nightingale and Ignaz Semmelweis successfully used handwashing and hygiene to stop infections from spreading in hospitals. A British surgeon called Joseph Lister began using chemicals known as **antiseptics** to kill microbes, making **operations far safer.**

GERM HERO

FLORENCE NIGHTINGALE

Founder of modern nursing. One of the first people to realize that hygiene and sanitation were powerful tools to stop the spread of infectious disease.

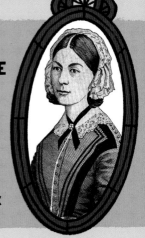

Even so, Pasteur's 'germ theory' was not believed straight away. In the mid-1800s, the most popular idea about the cause of infections was still an old idea from the Middle Ages—that smelly air or 'miasma' was to blame. It's not such a silly idea—places that smell bad and **smelly things** like rotten meat *are* linked with diseases. When they're cleaned up, diseases vanish too.

Germ theory was proved once and for all by Robert Koch, who showed that a disease called **anthrax** was caused by a specific type of bacteria.

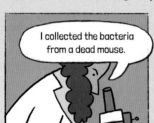

I collected the bacteria from a dead mouse.

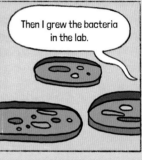

Then I grew the bacteria in the lab.

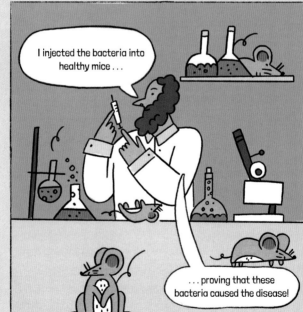

I injected the bacteria into healthy mice . . .

. . . proving that these bacteria caused the disease!

GERM HERO

ROBERT KOCH

German scientist who proved that germs cause disease, kick-starting a new science of tiny living things—microbiology!

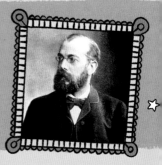

With the help of brilliant technicians such as Fanny Hesse, **microbiologists** developed new ways to grow and study these **tiniest** of living things in the lab. Koch realized that different **species** of bacteria have life cycles as different as those of lions and starfish, or frogs and fish. This explained how they caused so many different diseases and illnesses.

Kitasato Shibasaburō trained with Robert Koch. He studied the bacteria that caused tetanus and diphtheria and discovered that it wasn't the microbes themselves that caused the symptoms but **toxins** they released. Once he knew this, he was able to develop **antitoxins** to treat the illnesses.

Microbiologists **travelled the world**, identifying the microbes responsible for dozens of deadly diseases.

Working alongside Shibasaburō, Alexandre Yersin even managed to solve a mystery that had terrified the world for 700 years—identifying the bacteria that caused bubonic plague (page 13). He even invented an **antiserum** ('anti' at the beginning of a word means 'against') to treat patients. In the 1970s, the plague-causing bacteria were named *Yersinia pestis* in Yersin's honour.

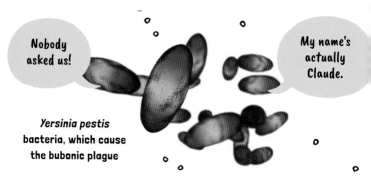

Yersinia pestis
**bacteria, which cause
the bubonic plague**

By the early 1900s, doctors and scientists knew that germs were pathogenic (disease-causing) microbes, capable of causing illness if they lived inside a plant, animal, or person. They knew these microbes had life cycles that helped pass them from person to person.

But many illnesses remained a mystery. When microbiologists studied samples of tissue from people infected with smallpox, measles, or influenza under a microscope, they couldn't see any microbes.

This suggested that there were even smaller germs yet to be discovered. These mysterious germs were named viruses, meaning **'poisonous slime'**. Were they extremely tiny bacteria? Or something else?

Once again, new technology led to the breakthrough. In 1939, an **electron microscope** finally let scientists see viruses—the smallest germs of all. Since then, scientists such as June Almeida have developed better methods to study viruses using electron microscopes that can magnify millions rather than thousands of times.

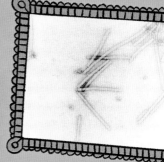

Tobacco mosaic virus was the first virus ever detected.

GERM HERO

JUNE ALMEIDA

In the 1960s, Almeida was the first person to see many viruses, including rubella and coronaviruses.

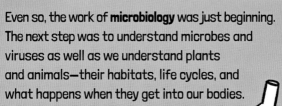

Even so, the work of **microbiology** was just beginning. The next step was to understand microbes and viruses as well as we understand plants and animals—their habitats, life cycles, and what happens when they get into our bodies.

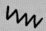

Chapter 3

Meet the Germs

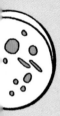

When Antonie van Leeuwenhoek first marvelled at the microbes living on his teeth (page 17), he could tell they were living creatures. At first he called them 'little animals', and there are plenty of tiny animals, such as fleas, that can only be seen in detail with the help of a microscope. But van Leeuwenhoek soon realized microbes are totally different life forms.

Microbes are far smaller than fleas. They are the smallest living things on our planet. They are far simpler than fleas too. A flea's body is made up of billions of **cells**, but each microbe is made up of just one cell.

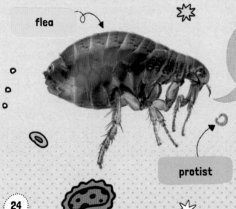

flea

I'm so much **more** complicated.

In real life, this flea is twenty times longer than this protist.

protist

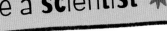

✳ Speak like a scientist ✳

CELL

Cells are the building blocks of living things. Your body is made up of trillions of cells, all doing different jobs. A single cell might seem too small to be a complete living thing, but cells are like miniature cities, with zones that carry out different tasks—from controlling and powering the cell to building and transporting chemicals.

Just as there are millions of different types (or species) of plants and animals, there are millions of different types of germs, with different habitats and life cycles. They fall into four main groups.

TYPES OF GERM	
bacteria	protists
fungi	viruses

Bacteria, fungi, and protists are all types of **single-celled** microbes. Viruses are even smaller and simpler than microbes. They don't have any cells at all. Let's take a closer look at each group.

Bacteria

Bacteria are the simplest microbes. Each **bacterium** is made up of one cell, and this cell is more basic than the cells of other living things. Despite this, bacteria are the most successful living things on Earth! Around 10,000 species have been discovered and named so far, but scientists estimate there could be millions.

The first bacteria seen by humans were rod-shaped, so were named after the Greek word **bakterion** meaning 'little stick'. But there are bacteria shaped like spheres, commas, and spirals too.

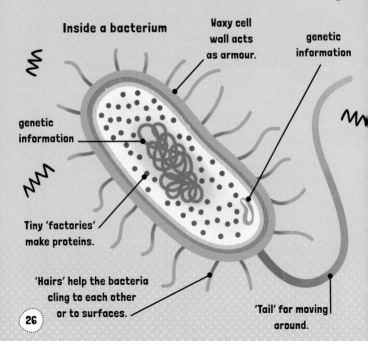

Inside a bacterium

Waxy cell wall acts as armour.

genetic information

genetic information

Tiny 'factories' make proteins.

'Hairs' help the bacteria cling to each other or to surfaces.

'Tail' for moving around.

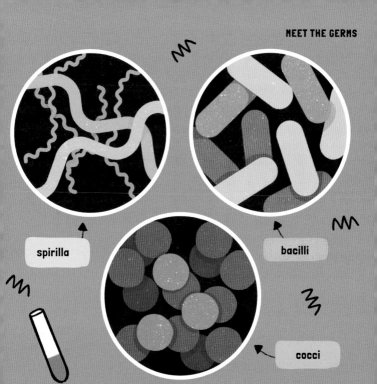

spirilla

bacilli

cocci

Over the last 3.5 billion years, different species of bacteria have **adapted** to live almost anywhere, from hot volcanoes to frozen Arctic snow. A few species share the superpower of plants—the ability to capture light energy and make their own food. Some **extremophile** bacteria can even capture the toxic chemicals spewed from superheated vents deep beneath the ocean and reassemble them into food. But most bacteria live in gentler environments and must find food ready-made. They do not have mouths. They simply soak up nutrients from their surroundings!

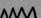

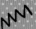

Bacteria and our bodies

Bacteria are surprisingly social. You might spot large groups living around the plughole of a sink or on your tongue. We are discovering that bacteria can share information using chemical signals and work together to control their community!

Bacteria like to live alongside larger living things too. Plants, animals, and people contain hundreds of different habitats where bacteria can survive and thrive.

Bacteria reproduce by splitting in two—making copies of themselves. Some species of bacteria do this so quickly that their population can grow **exponentially** (the larger the population gets, the faster it multiplies).

Some bacteria multiply so fast there can be up to **30 billion cells in a single millilitre of liquid** before they start to run out of food and space!

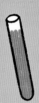

Some bacteria become harmful when they multiply very quickly, as they overwhelm our body's natural defences and begin using up the nutrients needed by our own cells. Others are harmful because they produce substances called **toxins**.

However, most bacteria are harmless to humans. In fact, trillions of bacteria share our bodies and we barely notice (see page 28)! Only around a tenth of the species of bacteria we have discovered so far are capable of causing humans harm, and fewer than 100 species are able to cause **infectious diseases** that can pass from person to person.

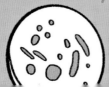

Most of us are lovely when you get to know us.

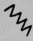

Fungi

It's easy to see a mushroom without a microscope! Many fungi (such as mushrooms or moulds) are made up of more than one cell. But the 135,000 known species of fungi include some single-celled microbes, such as **yeasts**. Some of these can be germs. Larger fungi also produce microscopic **spores**, and some of these are germs.

Inside the cell of a fungus

Even single-celled fungi are more complex than bacteria. Their cells are more like the cells of plants and animals.

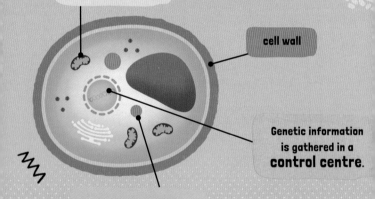

Tiny 'power stations' **unlock** the energy in food.

cell wall

Genetic information is gathered in a **control centre**.

tiny **'factories'** where proteins are made

Like bacteria, fungi are found almost everywhere. Many different types live in soil, where they feed on dead plants and animals. Others live closely together with plants, each helping the other to survive. However, some fungi are **parasites**—taking their **host's** nutrients, water, and energy but giving nothing back.

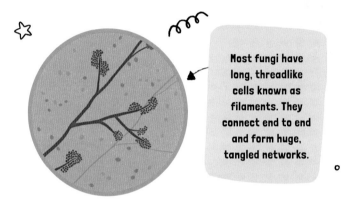

Most fungi have long, threadlike cells known as filaments. They connect end to end and form huge, tangled networks.

Fungi may harm their hosts by producing toxins or by using up too much of the resources that a plant or animal needs for itself. Fungal spores can also harm humans by triggering conditions such as asthma.

Fungi cause very few deadly infections in humans. However, many fungi are **serious pests** to plants. When fungi **infect crops** or grow on stored food and spoil it, they can cause food shortages, which can be just as deadly as diseases.

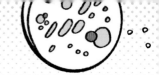

Protists

Protists are the third type of microbes that can also be germs—and are the most varied group of living things. They feed, move, live, and reproduce in thousands of different ways.

Although most protists are made up of just one cell, they are more like plants or animals than bacteria. Many have tails or hairs to help them move around. Some build hard shells. Others can make their own food using the energy in sunlight. Some even cluster together to make bigger living organisms, such as slime moulds that creep along the ground, gobbling up bacteria!

This species is known as **dog vomit slime mould.**

That is GROSSLY unfair!

Protists do have one thing in common: they all like to live in watery habitats, including inside plants and animals. Some are parasites that cause plant diseases and damage crops.

DISEASES CAUSED BY PROTISTS

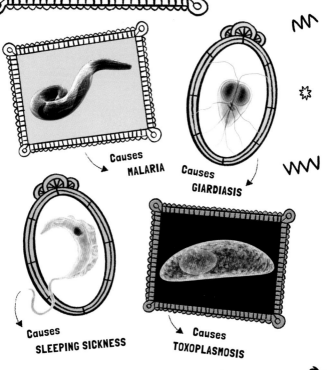

Causes
MALARIA

Causes
GIARDIASIS

Causes
SLEEPING SICKNESS

Causes
TOXOPLASMOSIS

Malaria is one of the world's deadliest diseases. It is caused by a type of protist called plasmodium. Instead of reproducing by simply splitting in two (as bacteria do), they have **very complicated life cycles,** which involve infecting two different animals: humans and mosquitoes.

Viruses

Viruses are the smallest, simplest, and most common germs. Up to 100,000 bacteria would fit on the head of a pin, but viruses are so small that up to a million would fit in the same space! In fact, most of the bacteria living on or in us are themselves infected with viruses known as **phages**.

bacterium

phage (virus)

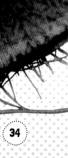

Colds, influenza, chickenpox, measles, hepatitis, warts, **gastroenteritis**, cold sores, and Covid–19 are all illnesses caused by viruses.

There are even viruses that transform healthy human and animal cells into **cancer** cells, which then start growing out of control.

Scientists still aren't sure if viruses count as living things. Viruses are not cells. They are just bits of **genetic information** wrapped in a protective coat. They have no way to feed, move, get energy from food, or make **proteins**. But they can hijack living cells and turn them into virus factories!

Inside a virus particle

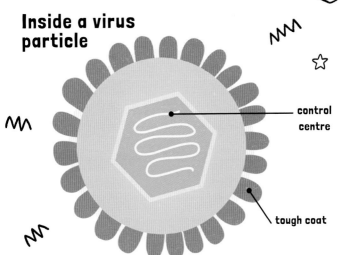

control centre

tough coat

Once a virus gets into a cell, the cell follows the genetic instructions provided by the virus and makes thousands of new viruses. These new viruses burst free, often destroying the host cell in the process, before infecting thousands of new host cells. The cycle starts again.

Only a few thousand types of virus have been studied and named so far, but we know they can infect every type of living thing, including other types of germs! For example, bacteria that cause diphtheria and cholera are only harmful because they are infected by phages, which give the bacteria cells the instructions to make toxins. Without these viruses, the bacteria are harmless.

If this sounds weird, wait till you hear that around 8% of your genetic information comes from ancient viruses! These viruses carried the genetic information for building proteins that turned out to be useful for humans. They became a permanent part of the human **genome** millions of years ago!

Sadly, viruses don't leave **fossils** behind, so no one is sure how long they have been around. Perhaps they existed before cells did. Or perhaps they evolved more recently from microbes.

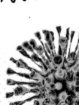

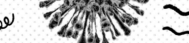

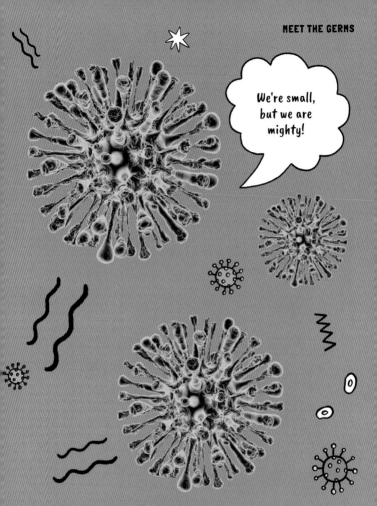

We're small, but we are mighty!

Either way, viruses have been incredibly successful. They are found everywhere on Earth in numbers too big to imagine. An individual virus may be impossible to see, but together the world's viruses are estimated to weigh three times more than all humans put together!

37

Chapter 4

How Do Germs Spread?

Some microbes only become germs when they find their way from their usual habitats into our bodies. In this new habitat, they can cause harm.

For example, fungi known as **dermatophytes** normally live in soil. But if they come into contact with our skin, they make themselves at home—they love warm, damp places like the gaps between toes on sweaty feet! The fungi are happy in their new habitat but our feet are not. The waste products the fungi produce make our skin swell and itch. We call this **infection** 'athlete's foot'.

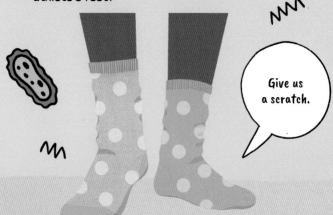

Give us a scratch.

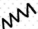

Friend or foe?

Sometimes, germs invade from a different part
of our own bodies. Our skin is covered in lots of
different colonies of **staphylococcus** bacteria.
They do no harm unless their habitat (our skin)
gets out of balance, when they can
suddenly start multiplying and
cause skin infections. And if
certain species get into a
person's blood or lungs, they can
cause life-threatening illnesses
such as sepsis or pneumonia.

We are covered in microscopic
fungi too, which also cause
infections. The yeast candida is a
fungus that normally **lives on our
skin** and in openings like our mouths and
throats. If the conditions inside our mouth or throat
change, the candida can multiply so much it causes
an infection known as oral thrush.

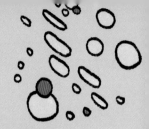

Passengers on food

Some germs live happily in animals without causing trouble but cause chaos if they get into humans—often as passengers on our food. Salmonella bacteria normally live in the intestines of animals, including farm animals and pets. These bacteria are such tough survivors that a piece of raw chicken, an egg, or a piece of cheese made from unpasteurized milk may contain live salmonella—even after hours spent in lorries, shops, fridges, and freezers!

Vegetables grown in fields fertilized by **animal manure** may also carry salmonella bacteria. If we don't wash or cook the food well enough to destroy the bacteria, they can cause an illness with fever, tummy pain, and **diarrhoea**.

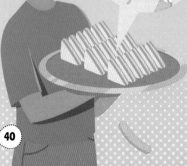

In some conditions, bacteria can multiply quickly on foods. But a few simple steps—storing, washing, and cooking—stops our food becoming a festival for microbes!

Typhoid Mary

The story of Mary Mallon helped scientists work out how easily infections caused by germs could be spread through food. Mary's body carried a type of salmonella bacteria that causes the disease typhoid. Although the bacteria never made her ill, Mary passed the bacteria to more than fifty people because she rarely washed her hands while working as a cook. In the late 1800s and early 1900s, people didn't yet understand the importance of handwashing.

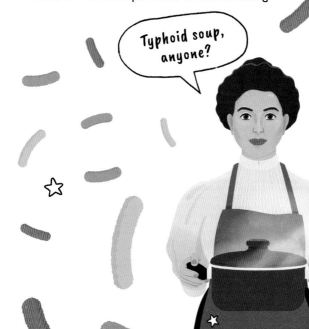

Typhoid soup, anyone?

41

Getting crowded

A single microbe or virus can't harm a plant or animal on its own. But, like all living things, bacteria, fungi, and protists reproduce. Viruses do too—by **tricking other cells** into making copies of them. A huge colony of germs begins to use up the nutrients and resources that their host needs to stay healthy. Germs may also harm large numbers of cells directly.

But germs can't keep multiplying forever in one host. Eventually they either:

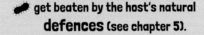 run out of **space** and nutrients

kill the **plant or animal**

get beaten by the host's natural **defences** (see chapter 5).

Some germs solve this problem by spreading to a new host before it's too late. These are the germs that cause **infectious diseases**—diseases that can be passed from one living thing to another.

Many germs are brilliant at causing symptoms that help them spread. The rhinoviruses that cause common colds turn a human being into a virus production and launch system!

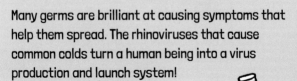

Viruses infect nose and throat cells.

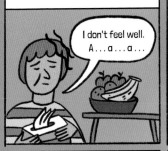

Droplets of snot rush out at up to 160 kph.

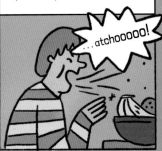

Each droplet is packed with millions of viruses. People breathe them in.

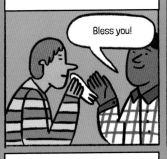

Some droplets land on food or surfaces and stick to people's hands.

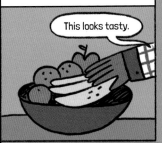

Viruses find themselves in a new host.

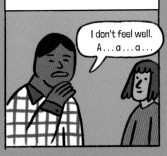

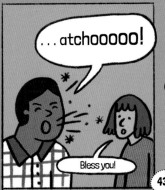

43

Sneezes spread diseases

Coughing and sneezing are the most common ways that germs find a new host. Colds and flu spread like this, as well as infections such as Covid-19, meningitis, and tuberculosis (TB).

Some germs find a more dramatic route out of our bodies. Rotaviruses infect and harm the cells that line our intestines, causing vomiting and diarrhoea packed with viruses. If infected people don't wash their hands after using the loo, or if the fluids find their way into water that people use to swim, bathe in, or drink, the viruses spread easily to other people.

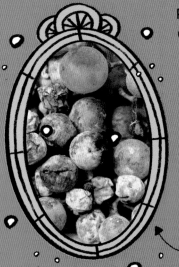

Plants don't sneeze or get diarrhoea, so many of the germs that affect plants are spread by **spores**. These are special cells produced by microbes. They spread in wind and water or are carried on the bodies of insects. When a spore finds itself in a good habitat, it grows into a new microbe.

The spores made by the fungal disease called powdery mildew make grapes look dusty.

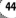

Other germs are too fragile to survive outside their host. They can only be spread by direct contact—when blood or other body fluids mix. Some germs take advantage of another animal's life cycle to find a new host. For example, if a rabbit has a bacterial infection called treponematosis and it mates with another rabbit, it can pass on the bacteria. Diseases that spread like this are known as sexually transmitted infections (STIs) in animals or **sexually transmitted diseases (STDs)** in humans.

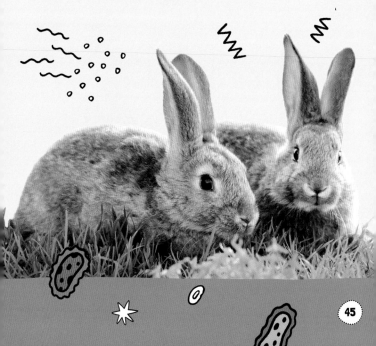

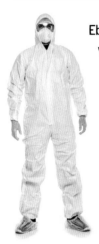

Ebola virus is one of the deadliest human viruses. It infects the cells of a patient's blood vessels, and a single drop of infected blood can contain up to a billion viruses. The viruses are also found in a person's sweat. If someone touches the patient, or their clothes or bedding, the virus can get into their body through any tiny cuts on their skin. Medics treating Ebola virus patients must wear very good **personal protective equipment (PPE)** to stay safe.

The need for contact means Ebola doesn't spread as quickly and easily as many germs do. During an outbreak of Ebola in West Africa in 2014, each patient passed the infection on to between 1.5 and 2.5 people. Scientists say it has an **R_0** ['R nought'] of 1.5 to 2.5.

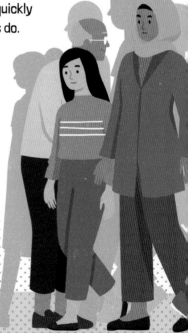

✱ Speak like a scientist ✱

R_0

R_0 is short for the 'reproduction number' of a disease. It describes how many new people an infected person is likely to pass the disease on to—how easily the disease spreads. Measles spreads very easily—it can have an R_0 as high as 18, meaning each infected person can infect up to 18 others. Then each of those 18 people will infect up to 18 others, and so on.

If one person with measles infects 18 people, then each of those infects another 18, that's 325 people with measles!

Taxis for germs

Long before people knew what germs were, they knew that staying at a distance from ill people could stop disease from spreading (page 12). This breaks the chain of infection. Germs that can't survive in the big bad world on their own are at risk of **becoming extinct!** Some fragile germs get around this problem by hitching a ride between humans or animals.

Biting insects such as mosquitoes make brilliant germ taxis—or **vectors**. The females of these small animals spend their time looking for larger animals to bite in order to get the nutrients needed to produce eggs. They can move or fly long distances and land on these animals undetected. When they bite or scratch an animal, any germs they picked up from their last meal get transferred to the new host.

The germs may need to live in very different ways in each host. If they make the insects sick, they won't get their **free ride.** As a result, protists that rely on insect vectors often have very complicated life cycles. This explains why the malaria-causing protist plasmodium has so many different costume changes (page 33).

1. Infected mosquito bites a person to get the nutrients it needs to produce eggs. Protists in its saliva pass into the person's blood.

7. Protists change again, making their way from the mosquito's gut to its salivary glands.

2. Protists make themselves at home in liver cells and change.

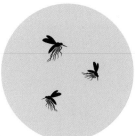

3. Thousands burst out into the person's blood.

6. Mosquito slurps up blood and protists.

4. Protists get into red blood cells, feed on proteins, and change into different forms.

5. Now the person feels very ill, so they rest in bed—an easy target for biting mosquitoes.

Perfect conditions for germs

Humans live in ways that give germs a helping hand. We crowd close together in cities and towns, and gather in large groups to learn, work, and have fun, and this gives germs opportunities to spread easily from person to person. When we travel for work or holidays, germs jet around the world alongside us.

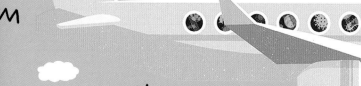

We produce food by keeping herds or flocks of the same animal, and planting crops in huge fields. This gives germs opportunities to spread easily from animal to animal or plant to plant. We also intrude into the habitats of other animals, bringing ourselves into contact with new germs. Thousands of years ago, the ancestors of the microbes that cause measles, mumps, and whooping cough were germs that only affected animals. Today **zoonoses** (infectious diseases that jump from animals to humans) are still the main source of new human diseases.

Dumping fertilizer, sewage, and other types of pollution can change **ecosystems** and throw them **off balance**, giving microbes such as algae and bacteria a chance to multiply and cause problems.

Knowing about germs is the first step in working out how to break chains of infection, but as scientists such as Carlos Chagas recognized, the spread of disease can't just be blamed on microbes and insects. Making sure everyone has good living conditions and access to healthcare and education can be just as important.

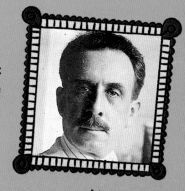

GERM HERO

CARLOS CHAGAS

He discovered the protist that causes deadly Chagas disease and showed how it spreads from person to person.

Chapter 5

Natural Defences

Human hands are germ magnets! They produce natural oils that help microbes cling on to our skin and pick up millions of microbes every day—which may include some harmful germs. We then use those same hands to rub our eyes, touch our mouths, pick our noses, or handle food. One study found that we touch our faces twenty-three times an hour! In a world full of microbes and germs, why don't we get ill all the time?

The answer lies in our own **extraordinary adaptations.** Every plant, animal, and person has natural defences against germs—defences that have evolved over millions of years of sharing a planet with microbes and viruses.

The first layer of defence is about keeping microbes out. It's a highly **effective armour** of snot, sweat, tears, and earwax!

Earwax traps invading germs. It's also waterproof, keeping your ear canal dry so water-loving microbes are less likely to set up camp.

Sweat and tears contain salts and proteins that harm germs.

Saliva contains natural antiseptics.

Sticky mucus traps microbes before they can get to our lungs. We swallow up to 1.5 litres of mucus every day!

Most swallowed microbes are destroyed by strong stomach acid.

Skin is a waterproof, germproof barrier. Cuts are quickly sealed with scabs.

Immune defences

If germs do get through your snotty, sweaty, waxy outer armour, your **immune system** is ready to track down and destroy harmful microbes and viruses inside your body too. It is your personal army, made up of different types of cells.

General defences

White blood cells are always on duty and will target ANYTHING they don't recognize. They include **macrophages** (meaning **'big eaters'** from the Greek word for devour), which chase germs, engulf them, and destroy them! You know they're at work if a cut or infected area is red and swollen.

White blood cell

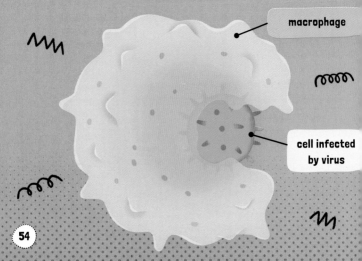

macrophage

cell infected by virus

Specific defences

These white blood cells work more slowly but very effectively. When they come across a germ (or infected cell), they tag it with special chemicals called **antibodies**. Each type of antibody is specially made to latch on to a specific chemical, known as an **antigen**, on a specific germ. Once latched on, the antibodies act as a big flag that helps your general defences track down the right cells and viruses to kill!

antibodies

virus

The first time a germ gets into your body, it takes your white blood cells a few days to learn to make the right antibodies. But the antibodies stay in your blood after an infection. Next time that same antigen appears in your body, your antibodies and white blood cells **spring into action** straight away. This 'memory' means the germs are destroyed before they can multiply and make you ill. You now have **immunity** to that germ!

☀ Speak like a scientist ☀

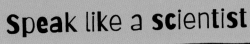

IMMUNITY

When your immune system is able to fight off an infection caused by a certain germ so quickly that you don't get any symptoms.

Give your body a helping hand

Every plant, animal, and microbe has some kind of defence system against invading germs. Many also behave in a way that helps to protect them from germs.

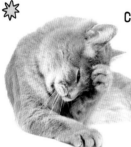

Cats have an instinct to lick cuts and scratches, delivering antimicrobial saliva. Cats even have long spines on their tongues to **comb** saliva deep into their fur.

On top of these natural defences and behaviours, humans have developed other ways to help us live alongside germs without being harmed.

The most important of these is also the simplest— washing. As Florence Nightingale discovered, washing our hands for at least twenty seconds is the best way to vanquish the millions of microbes and viruses that collect on our skin during **a busy day.** Soap is an important part of washing. It breaks up skin oils so they can be rinsed away, carrying germs with them. It may also break up some germs themselves!

Hands should be **washed with soap:**

☀ before and after preparing food/eating

☀ after using the toilet

☀ after being near animals or animal waste

☀ after coughing, sneezing, blowing (and picking) your nose

☀ if you are ill or have been around ill people.

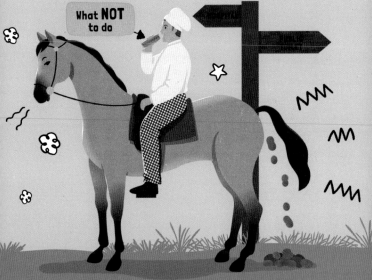

What **NOT** to do

People noticed the power of handwashing long before they knew germs existed. Today we should be experts. But study after study shows that most people do not wash their hands often enough or well enough—even after using the loo!

Kitchen battleground

Food is one of the main routes for germs to get into our bodies, so storing, washing, and cooking food correctly are also important ways in which we can stop germs spreading.

The **pasteurization** process (developed by Louis Pasteur himself, page 18) involves heating liquid foods gently to destroy disease-causing microbes without cooking the food. Most microbes we find on food are killed at temperatures above 70°C.

Pasteurization means we can store milk, fruit juice, and dairy products made with pasteurized milk for longer periods in the fridge. Some solid foods are also 'pasteurized', using microwaves or other radiation instead of heat energy.

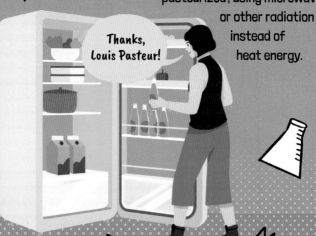

Thanks, Louis Pasteur!

Keeping food very cold can also **stop germs** from growing. In a fridge or freezer, some microbes will die, but others are just on pause and start to multiply again once they get warm. This is one reason we cook many foods before we eat them—so that harmful germs are killed by heat. It's also why handwashing is so important in kitchens, especially after handling raw meat or fish.

If foods are eaten raw, it's important to **wash them first.** Most of the microbes found on fruit and vegetables are harmless, but sometimes germs lurk in the soil in which they are grown or in the manure used to fertilize them.

Care is also taken while our foods are still on the farm. For example, vets help farmers to reduce the bacteria in and on animals farmed for food.

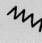

Sanitation sensation

Which technology has done most to help humans live longer lives on a planet packed with germs? **Is it the refrigerator? The oven? Soap?**

> Or ... the flushing toilet?

Public sanitation systems carry waste water and sewage away from our homes and into sewers, keeping it away from sources of drinking water. The water is then thoroughly cleaned before being released back into the environment.

In water treatment plants, billions of bacteria and protists are hard at work cleaning the water we use for our everyday lives and manufacturing. Friendly bacteria feed on polluting chemicals dissolved in the water, converting them into biogas (a mixture of the gases carbon dioxide and methane), which can be burned to produce electricity. Harmful bacteria, such as salmonella and *E. coli*, perish in the tough conditions. Hungry protists also hunt down bacteria to eat. Later, both types of microbes are removed from the water by filters.

In many countries, sanitation systems work so well that **we take them for granted.** But 4.5 billion people (more than half the world's population) still live without access to a toilet, putting them at risk of diseases such as cholera, dysentery, and typhoid fever.

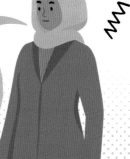

Tackling germs doesn't always mean inventing fancy new technologies or medicines. It means ensuring that everyone has fair access to the technologies that already exist.

Chapter 6

Medicines Versus Microbes

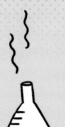

Our natural defences are good at keeping germs at bay. But germs are always adapting, evolving new ways to get past our outer defences and foil our immune systems. For example, the bacteria that cause tuberculosis and the virus that causes HIV/AIDS infect the cells of our immune system, making them very hard for our bodies to destroy. Some people are also naturally more vulnerable to germs than others.

Since ancient times, people have tried to invent medicines that give our bodies a helping hand.

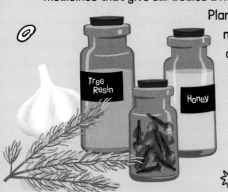

Plants have their own natural defences against microbes, so plants have been used as sources of microbe-killing chemicals.

Tree Resin

Honey

Ancient peoples found that other natural substances, such as honey and tree resin, have antimicrobial properties if they are smeared on wounds, too.

Developing medicines that can be used to kill microbes inside a person's body is harder. Many germ-killing substances, such as antiseptics, would harm our own cells too if we ate or drank them, causing nasty side effects. Again, plants have often provided solutions for scientists who looked closely enough. In Hawaii in the early 1900s, Alice Ball worked out how to turn oil from chaulmoogra trees into a medicine that could be used to treat Hansen's disease (also known as leprosy) safely.

Chaulmoogra

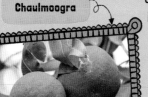

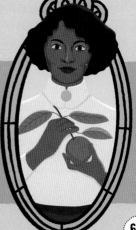

GERM HERO

ALICE BALL

Alice unlocked the chemistry of plants to make medicines.

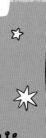

Developing new medicines can be very difficult and often relies on **trial and error.** By the time Tu Youyou began looking for cures for malaria in the 1960s, 240,000 different chemicals had already been tested and none had worked. She looked for clues through hundreds of ancient Chinese medical books and found a tiny note about sweet wormwood. This led Youyou to track down a chemical in the plant called artemisinin, which she developed into a medicine that has saved millions of lives.

There are many stories like this, and they are one reason why it's so important to protect Earth's millions of different living things. It's like a library full of secrets we haven't yet discovered, including new drugs to treat infections.

GERM HERO

TU YOUYOU

Tu Youyou developed a medicine to treat malaria, a disease that kills millions of people every year.

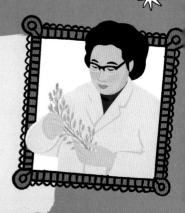

Germ versus germ

In recent years, the world has been focused on ways to vanquish viruses. But for most of human history, disease-causing bacteria were the **biggest threat**. Even a small scratch could let harmful bacteria into a person's body and prove deadly. This changed in the 1940s, thanks to the discovery of **antibiotics**.

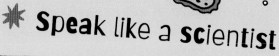

Speak like a scientist

ANTIBIOTICS

Antibiotics are substances produced by microbes to keep bacteria at bay. Alexander Fleming discovered the first antibiotic, penicillin, in 1928. It is made by mould and stops bacteria from building their protective cell walls (page 26), so they explode! It doesn't harm humans or animals because our cells don't have cell walls. Howard Florey and Ernst Chain turned penicillin into a medicine, and since then it has saved millions of lives.

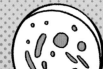

Penicillin works on lots of different bacteria—including the ones that cause deadly diseases such as pneumonia and diphtheria—but it doesn't work on them all. Scientists including Selman Waksman, Elizabeth Bugie, and Albert Schatz began searching for more of these **'miracle' medicines** and found them in soil. They spent years collecting thousands of different **species** of streptomycetes (a type of bacteria that live in soil), working out which chemicals these bacteria use against their enemies, then checking that the chemicals were safe for humans and other animals. Streptomycetes are the source of more than half the antibiotics used as medicines. They can fight the bacteria that cause tuberculosis, typhoid, and cholera.

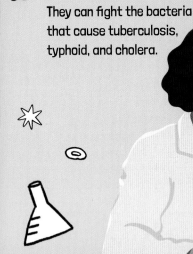

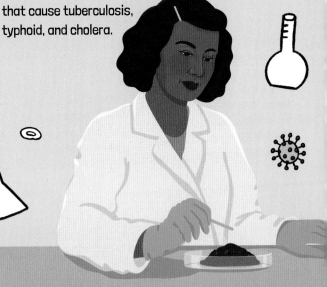

GERM HERO

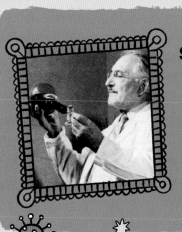

SELMAN WAKSMAN

He invented the word antibiotic (meaning 'against life') and led the discovery of hundreds of new antibiotics, including streptomycin.

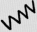

In 1950, half of the world's population died before they were 46 years old. By 2015, the average life expectancy had increased to 72 years. Antibiotics were a huge part of this increase in average life span and are still the main weapon we have against harmful bacteria. But, as Fleming himself predicted almost as soon as he discovered penicillin, **bacteria are fighting back** (page 78).

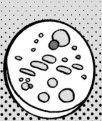

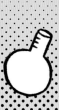

Vaccination

Antibiotics treat infections and diseases caused by bacteria, but they cannot treat viral diseases such as colds, influenza, or Covid-19. Antiviral medicines have been developed, and some have been very successful. But our ultimate weapon against diseases caused by viruses (and many other infectious diseases) is **vaccination**.

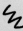

The basics of vaccination were discovered long before anyone knew what a germ was. In China and India, people worked out that exposing children to the powdered scabs or pus of smallpox victims gave them a mild form of the disease but protected them from catching it later in life. The method spread, and in Europe people even held 'smallpox parties', where parents sent their children to catch it on purpose. But it was risky, and not everyone took part, so smallpox still spread.

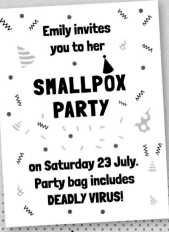

Emily invites you to her

SMALLPOX PARTY

on Saturday 23 July.
Party bag includes
DEADLY VIRUS!

In the 1700s, the doctor Edward Jenner noticed that farmworkers who had recovered from a similar (but less serious) disease called cowpox seemed to be protected from smallpox. He tested this idea by infecting a 9-year-old with cowpox on purpose. Two months later, he did something that would be **unthinkable today** and dabbed a scratch on the boy's arm with pus from a smallpox patient. This huge risk paid off—the boy didn't get ill. Jenner called his new preventative treatment 'vaccination' after the Latin for cowpox (*vacca* means cow in Latin).

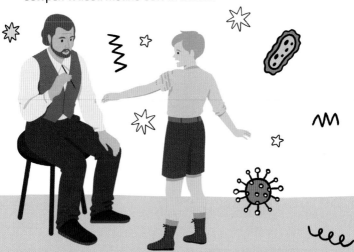

Jenner didn't know it at the time, but the **antibodies** made by the boy's immune system to fight off cowpox also worked against the smallpox virus. Vaccination against smallpox has been so successful that by 1980, there were no more cases anywhere in the world. It was the first virus to be **totally eradicated** and wiped out!

At first it seemed impossible to repeat this with diseases that didn't have a less serious form. But in the 1800s, Louis Pasteur worked out how to make artificial vaccines. He heated deadly microbes to make them weaker before injecting them into animals. The germs were too weak to make the animals ill, but their immune systems still learned how to recognize the antigens. Future invaders stood no chance!

Vaccines are still made using dead or weakened microbes and viruses. In many countries, babies and young children are given vaccinations that give them lifelong protection from dozens of diseases that were once common and deadly—such as tetanus, measles, whooping cough, polio, and diphtheria. As we've learned that some cancers are linked to microbes, we have even been able to develop vaccines that protect against these particular cancers.

Vaccination saves **millions of lives** every year, but it's not possible to create a vaccine that gives lasting protection for every disease. Some germs, such as influenza viruses, have a way to get around an immune system that never forgets.

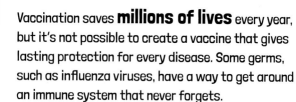

These viruses change their outer coats often, which also changes their antigens. Each time our immune system encounters flu, it has to relearn how to **fight it.** And the vaccines we have for flu have to be continually updated to keep up with these new influenza variants.

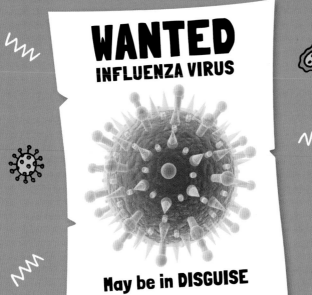

WANTED
INFLUENZA VIRUS

May be in DISGUISE

Vaccination is not the only way we can give our immune systems a **helping hand.** Eating healthily, exercising, getting enough sleep, and taking steps to decrease stress are very important too.

New technologies

New technologies such as genomics speed up the process of developing vaccines and treatments. Studying the genomes of microbes gives us clues about how to tackle them. Within months of the first Covid-19 cases, teams of scientists around the world had studied the genomes of different strains of this coronavirus. They used what they found out to help develop vaccines against the disease.

Speak like a scientist

GENOMICS

Genomics is an area of science that studies the genetic information carried inside every living thing. This information is known as the plant, animal, or microbe's genome, and controls many aspects of its development.

Genomics helps doctors to predict which vaccines and medicines will work against which germs and to tailor medicines to suit individual patients.

Genomics also helps us to diagnose diseases more quickly. Instead of having to find microbes in a patient, grow them in the lab, and peer at them through a microscope, we can detect tiny amounts of the unique genetic information belonging to each type of germ. We can also detect these tiny traces in waste water in a town or city's sewage systems too, which can help to monitor and control disease epidemics.

Genomics has also helped us understand how microbes adapt and evolve resistance to antibiotics and vaccinations so quickly.

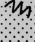

Medicines and vaccinations can seem miraculous—but they can't beat germs on their own. Just as some human behaviours help germs spread, changing behaviour can be a powerful way to break **chains of infection.** It can help to prevent diseases from happening in the first place. This is done through education and through **public health** communication.

- Finding out how to keep your immune system healthy.

- Learning how different germs spread, and how to avoid them.

- Learning why it's so important to take up vaccinations.

- Learning the right way to use medicines and methods of protecting ourselves from germs.

Can **words and education** really help tackle disease? Public health experts, such as **Quarraisha Abdool Karim**, know that it's not just about dropping information in front of people. Tasked with tackling the spread of HIV/AIDS in South Africa, Karim began by listening carefully to the groups of people most affected by the virus. By understanding how they live, and gaining their trust and respect, she was able to design public health measures that taught people how to **protect themselves and others.**

GERM HERO

QUARRAISHA ABDOOL KARIM

Developed public health measures that helped stop the spread of HIV/AIDS.

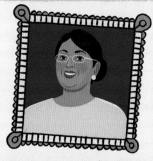

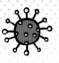

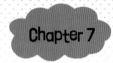

Chapter 7

Will We Ever Have a World Without Germs?

During the 20th and early 21st centuries, our relationship with germs was revolutionized! When the Covid-19 pandemic began, it was a sudden and shocking reminder of how human lives can be dominated by germs. Just 100 years ago, a tiny scratch or an infected tooth could be deadly. Serious illnesses such as measles were thought of as a normal part of childhood.

Today we know how germs cause harm, and how they spread. We have developed thousands of medicines, vaccinations, sanitation, and public health measures to help people live safely alongside germs. Vaccination has even vanquished some of the biggest killers of the last thousand years, such as smallpox and polio in humans and **rinderpest** in animals. In huge parts of the world, it is now normal to live a long, healthy life. Millions and millions of lives have been saved.

Speak like a scientist

RINDERPEST

Rinderpest was a viral disease that used to kill millions of cattle and other animals each year. In 2011, it became the first non-human disease to be eradicated thanks to a global effort using vaccination and other measures. It shows what is possible if countries work together to understand and implement scientific findings.

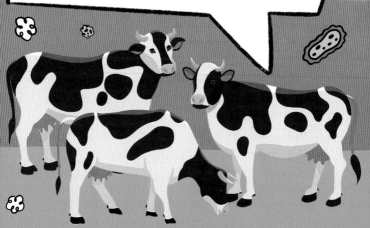

These successes have changed the world, but we will never rid the **planet of germs** altogether. It's proving very difficult to develop vaccines against some diseases, such as HIV/AIDS and malaria. They still kill millions of people around the world every year.

Myths and misconceptions can mean that people don't take up vaccinations that could one day save their lives. This is why there are still frequent outbreaks of measles that kill children, even though a vaccine for measles was invented in the 1960s.

Perhaps the biggest problem is that the medicines, vaccines, and healthcare that have been developed are not equally available to everyone. To tackle many of the world's **deadliest diseases**, we need to make sure that everyone can afford healthcare and live in safe and clean conditions.

Antimicrobial resistance

Microbes' short life cycles mean they adapt to changes in their environment far faster than plants and animals do. For example, any bacteria that just happen to be naturally resistant to antibiotics have a **huge advantage** when other bacteria are wiped out by a dose of antibiotics. They get all the host's energy, nutrients, and space to themselves and reproduce quickly. A single survivor can grow into a vast colony with each new bacterium inheriting its ancestor's resistance. Bacteria speed up this process even more by sharing useful genetic information with each other!

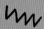

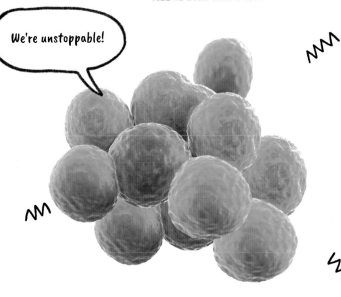

This problem—known as '**antimicrobial resistance**'—is one of the biggest issues facing the world. But small actions can help with this **big problem:**

🦠 only use antibiotics prescribed for you by a doctor

 🦠 always finish a course of antibiotics

🦠 don't ask for antibiotics for illnesses they can't treat, such as most coughs and colds.

Microbes on the menu

The more we learn about microbes, the more we find out how useful they can be in every area of life. Some microbes, such as yeasts, have cells remarkably similar to human cells, so yeasts have even helped doctors and scientists find out more about ourselves. They are also some of the microbes that help us make a huge range of everyday foods.

Bread is made using yeasts, which feed on sugar and produce the carbon dioxide gas that makes bread rise. This 'fermentation' is a vital step in producing other foods too. Foods like miso, dosa, pickles, chocolate, and some dairy products.

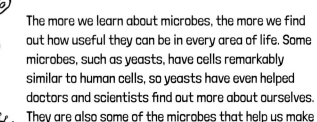

INGREDIENTS
FOR CHOCOLATE
• Cocoa • Milk
• Sugar • Yeasts
• Moulds • Bacteria

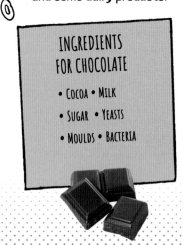

Chocolate can't be made without microbes. Yeasts, moulds, and bacteria must be left to feed on harvested cocoa beans for at least a week to give chocolate its very delicious flavour.

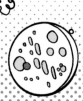

We also use microbes as tiny factories to produce food additives, vitamins, and medicines. Sometimes we collect substances naturally made by the microbes. Or we use genetic engineering to make microbes build useful proteins, such as human insulin, which is used to treat diabetes. It's a bit like farming—except the farmed creatures are microscopic and hang out in herds of billions!

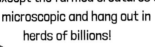
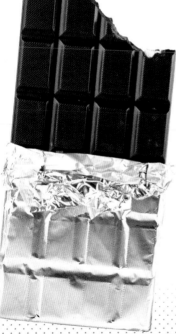
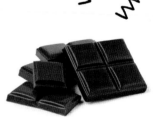

Microbiomes

Humans have been making things with microbes for thousands of years. But we are only just finding out how important they are for building our own bodies!

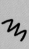

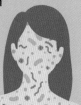

Our bodies contain **more microbial cells than human cells,** and that's not even counting the viruses.

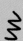

Altogether, our **microbiome** weighs **more than our brain**—and is just as important!

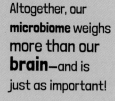

✳ Speak like a scientist ✳

> ## MICROBIOME
>
> The 'friendly' microbes and viruses that live inside a larger living thing.

We know lots about harmful microbes, or germs, but we're only just beginning to understand about the healthy microbes that make up the human microbiome. The research carried out by Abigail Salyers completely changed how we think about the microbes living in our bodies. They help digest our food, releasing nutrients we can't digest ourselves and building vitamins we can't build ourselves. They also protect us from invading germs just by being there. Our gut bacteria use up so much of the space and resources that dangerous microbes can't get a foothold. It's like having a tiny army to battle tiny invaders!

A third to a half of every poo you do is made of microbes, dead and alive!

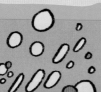

GERM HERO

ABIGAIL SALYERS

Microbiologist and 'mother of the microbiome', who also helped discover the tricks bacteria use to pass on antimicrobial resistance.

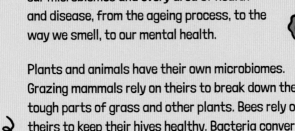

We are finding connections between our microbiomes and every area of health and disease, from the ageing process, to the way we smell, to our mental health.

Plants and animals have their own microbiomes. Grazing mammals rely on theirs to break down the tough parts of grass and other plants. Bees rely on theirs to keep their hives healthy. Bacteria convert nitrogen from the air into a form plants can use. Mycorrhizal fungi live on and inside roots, helping plants to absorb water and nutrients from the soil.

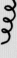

In fact, all **life on Earth** begins and ends with microbes. They were the first living things on the planet, and over billions of years they changed it by adding oxygen to the atmosphere. They created the conditions for animals and plants to evolve, and they are the ancestors of every living thing, including us!

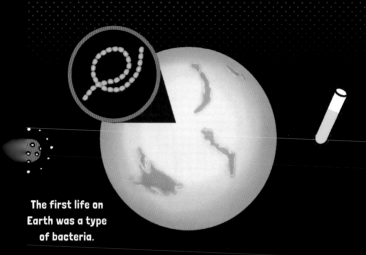

The first life on Earth was a type of bacteria.

The planet is still theirs. Every litre of seawater contains millions of microbes and billions of viruses. A handful of soil can contain more bacteria than there are humans on Earth. Every living thing is home to a huge community of microbes, which support life and continue their work even after their host dies. They become the first of the decomposers that break down dead plants and animals so that their building blocks can be recycled into new life.

Together, Earth's microbes are estimated to weigh forty times more than all its animals combined.

If all microbes did suddenly disappear, all other life on Earth would quickly follow

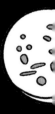

Chapter 8

The Future of Germs

Germs are here to stay but so is science.
Here are some of the questions that scientists
are hoping to answer in the future.

Will there be more pandemics and new diseases?

Although microbiologists were not
surprised by Covid-19, many people
were. In some countries, people had
got used to living without major
epidemics of infectious disease
thanks to vaccines and antimicrobials.
But the way humans live makes outbreaks
inevitable. There will be new diseases,
and they will most likely be **zoonoses**.
We interact with animals on farms, in
markets, in science, in the wild, and as pets.
Almost three quarters of all new human
infectious diseases in the past thirty
years began as germs in animals.

FUND VACCINE RESEARCH

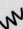

But not every zoonosis becomes an epidemic or pandemic. We can **stop this happening** by learning from the past, taking steps to prevent outbreaks, and acting quickly when they do occur. We can demand that our governments fund research into new antimicrobials and vaccines, act to improve living conditions, and make sure that everyone, no matter how much their family earns, can access healthcare.

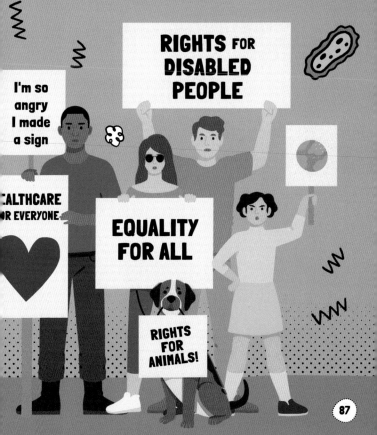

RIGHTS FOR DISABLED PEOPLE

I'm so angry I made a sign

~ALTHCARE ~R EVERYONE

EQUALITY FOR ALL

RIGHTS FOR ANIMALS!

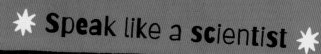

✳ Speak like a scientist ✳

ZOONOSES

Germs that jump from animal hosts to humans are called zoonoses. In the last fifty years these have included not only Covid-19 but Lyme disease (which began in deer and sheep), HIV/AIDS (which began in chimps and sooty mangabeys), SARS (which began in Chinese horseshoe bats), MERS (which began in camels), swine flu (which began in birds and pigs), and Zika virus (which began in rhesus monkeys). The virus that causes Covid-19 may have begun in bats too.

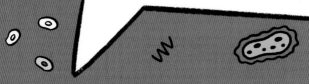

Can we harness germs to do good?

Humans have harnessed the unique ability of microbes in so many ways—such as making medicines and foods, cleaning waste water, and doing scientific research. We are also finding new ways to harness the 'superpowers' of microbes—including germs—to tackle big problems. For example, **plastic** waste usually takes hundreds of years to biodegrade, but certain microbes can digest it in weeks or months.

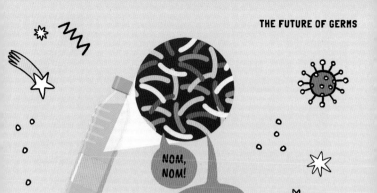

NOM, NOM!

DELICIOUS!

Understanding how microbes respond to global warming will be vital in tackling climate change too. As they live their lives, microbes both produce and use up greenhouse gases, such as carbon dioxide. Scientists have found that human activities are causing microbes to release more greenhouse gases than in the past.

Will we find germs on other planets?

If we do find life on other planets, it may well be in the form of microbes. But we also need to consider the impact of Earth's microbes on other worlds that we visit. The terrible diseases spread by European explorers and colonizers in the 15th and 16th centuries shows that germs can have a devastating effect if they are carried into new habitats. NASA's *Cassini* spacecraft was crashed into Saturn after its mission ended so it didn't **contaminate** Saturn's moons, some of the best places in our Solar System to hunt for life.

Can we get better at controlling germs?

We are getting better all the time. New technologies, such as microbe-killing materials, promise new ways to fight old germs. Researchers are also racing to find new anti-microbial medications and vaccinations. Discoveries about the links between our microbiomes (page 83), genomes, and our health will lead to new ways to fight and prevent disease.

But the Covid-19 pandemic has reminded us that simple actions—such as handwashing and social distancing—can also help us live more safely alongside germs.

Over the past 300 years, biologists have shown us how everything in nature is connected. Microbes and viruses—including germs— are at the heart of all our ecosystems. Every plant, animal, and human is an **ecosystem** full of microbes!

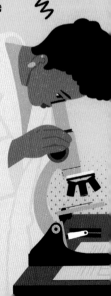

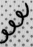

To tackle infection and disease, we need to think not just about germs but about the many complicated relationships between people, animals, plants, microbes, and the environments that we all share. This approach is known as One Health.

To germs, humans are just 7.8 billion potential hosts— one global community. To beat germs, we must act together—because germs don't have borders.

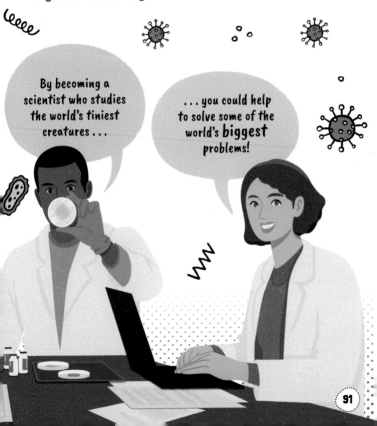

By becoming a scientist who studies the world's tiniest creatures . . .

. . . you could help to solve some of the world's **biggest** problems!

Glossary

adapt when a population of living things changes over time to become better suited to their environment

antibiotics substances produced by microbes to destroy or deter other microbes

antibodies proteins produced by a person's or animal's immune system that latch on to specific germs (or other substances that shouldn't be in the body) and flag them up to be destroyed

antigen a substance, such as a germ or a substance made by a germ, that makes an animal's immune system leap into action

antiseptics chemicals that stop microbes from growing

antiserum a medicine made from part of the blood, containing antibodies that will work against a specific disease

antitoxin a medicine containing antibodies that will work against a specific toxin

bacterium (plural bacteria) the word for a single bacterial cell

biodiversity the huge variety of living things in the world

cancer a type of disease caused by a person or animal's own cells that start growing out of control

cell smallest building block of a living thing

Chagas disease a very common disease in tropical Latin America.

contagious when a disease can be passed easily from person to person or animal to animal

decomposer a living thing that plays a part in decay

diarrhoea a symptom of some infectious diseases, with frequent and runny poo

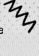

ecosystem a community of living things that all depend on one another

electron microscope a powerful microscope that allows scientists to magnify objects millions of times, using beams of electrons instead of light

epidemic when a disease spreads widely in a certain area

eradicated completely destroyed; no longer in the world

extremophile a living thing that thrives in extreme conditions that would kill most other living things

fluid a gas or liquid that can flow

fossils traces of organisms that lived on Earth long ago

gastroenteritis inflammation of the stomach and intestines, often caused by bacteria or viruses

genetic information the information carried inside every cell of a living thing (or by a virus) which tells the cells how to build proteins

genome the total genetic information carried inside every living thing (or virus)

host a person, plant, animal, or microbe with a microbe or virus living in or on them

hygiene taking steps to stay clean, or keep your environment clean

immune system your body's natural defence against invading germs

immunity lasting resistance to a disease, due to either a previous infection or a vaccination

infection a harmful invasion of germs

infectious disease a disease that can be passed from one living thing to another

microbes tiny living things that can only be seen with a microscope

microbiologist a scientist who studies microbes

microbiology the area of science interested in microbes

parasite an organism that lives in or on another organism, taking nutrients and other resources without giving anything back

pasteurization treating a food or other product to kill all or some of the microbes that would otherwise grow in it

pathogen a microbe or virus that can cause disease (also known as a germ)

pathogenic disease-causing

personal protective equipment (PPE) special clothes and equipment worn to protect a person from dangerous substances, such as germs

phage a virus that infects bacteria

proteins substances produced by all living cells that carry out different jobs as well as being building blocks of cells (and of viruses)

single-celled a living thing made up of just one cell

species a group of living things of the same kind

spore special cells produced by microbes to help them spread or reproduce

theory an idea about the best way to explain something

toxin a substance made by microbes that is harmful to other living things

trade when different countries buy from, and sell things to, each other

vaccination a dead or weakened form or a germ (or substance produced by that germ) that can teach a living thing's immune system how to recognize and fight the real thing

vector an animal that carries a disease-causing parasite from one animal or plant to another

yeast a type of single-celled fungus; there are many different species of yeasts

zoonoses infectious diseases that have jumped from animal hosts to humans

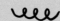

Index

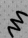

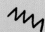